About Depression

By Bryan C. Price

Content

Dedication	Page 3
Prologue	Page 4
Chapter 1 – What is Depression	Page 8
Chapter 2 – Symptoms	Page 15
Chapter 3 – What you can say	Page 23
Chapter 4 – What not to say	Page 32
Chapter 5 – Treatment	Page 40
Chapter 6 – Three Deaths	Page 46
Epilogue	Page 50
Contributions and Thanks	Page 51

Dedication

I am dedicating this book to all victims that have taken their own lives, suffered suicidal thoughts and depression

Prologue

Winston Churchill called it the black dog. Many people suffer from different types of depression. Some are more severe than others. I have had to live with it for most of life. I have had difficulty to explain why I get depressed, so I decided I need to voice my thoughts to try understanding it in layman's terms. Phyciatrists can treat it chemically and Phycologists try getting it around by getting into your head, yet I don't understand it. As I get older I am finding it harder and harder to snap out of it. It is also taking longer to snap out of it as well. I tend to withdraw socially and try deal with it myself. When I was younger a day or two of conversations with myself would be enough for me to get out of it but now weeks go by and I really can't get out of it. The endless cycle of sadness and despair is really starting to take its toll to point that suicide is an option to end it all. Yet there is so much to live for and no reason to terminate my life. I have had enough of other people telling me what to do about it because I feel that they don't know what it is unless they suffer from depression themselves.

Quite frankly in my view no one is qualified to tell what I am thinking and no one is qualified to tell how I must deal with it. Every single time someone voices their opinion on how I must deal with it, it seems almost so cliché. There are other people out there with a similar mind set and this book is me having the courage to speak out and a platform for me to take what is going it in my head and letting other see and feel what I am thinking.

I undertook a journey of rediscovering myself by taking a five month sabbatical to write my memoirs. I under took not to look into a mirror for that period. At the end I had metamorphasized by losing almost 60kg from being 160kg to 100kg. While writing my memoirs

I experienced all the good and bad emotions that I was confronted with during the 50 years of my existence. I was on no medication. It was raw emotion that I felt that was not subdued or neutralized in any way. I was happy to feel happy, sad, and angry again.

Although it is dangerous not to medicate. I was in the privileged situation to allow myself the time I needed to heal and gather up my broken soul and piece the puzzle together again. After 18 Months of rediscovering myself I no longer have the dark thoughts that haunted me all my life.

I am able to commit to a relationship knowing that I carry no emotional baggage. I have incredible amounts of energy and look forward to every new day. I am able to think clearly.

I would like to share my positive experience with others. I can say that speaking out was the key to overcome depression. It is a taboo subject that people don't like talk about and I found people especially piers would judge you in a negative way. Mental health is a reality and affects people of all walks of life.

Having a bad day does not necessarily mean you are depressed. Everybody is entitled to a bad day. Depression not only affects the person but also the people around them as well.

Chapter One

"A healthy body will enable you to have a healthy mind"

What is depression?

Depression is a common and debilitating mood disorder. More than just sadness in response to life's struggles and setbacks, depression changes how you think, feel, and function in daily activities. It can interfere with your ability to work, study, eat, sleep, and enjoy life. The feelings of helplessness, hopelessness, and worthlessness can be intense and unrelenting, with little, if any, relief.

While some people describe depression as "living in a black hole" or having a feeling of impending doom, others feel lifeless, empty, and apathetic. Men in particular can feel angry and restless. No matter how you experience depression, left untreated it can become a serious health condition. But it's important to remember that feelings of helplessness and hopelessness are symptoms of depression—not the reality of your situation. There are plenty of powerful self-help steps you can take to lift your mood, overcome depression, and regain your joy of life.

Many people struggle to understand depression. What makes it difficult for them is that when they become depressed, there is a visible reason like an illness or the loss of a job. So, it can be difficult to comprehend why it doesn't work that way for other people. Why would someone be depressed if everything in their life is good?

What Causes Depression

The reason is that depression can be caused by a defect within the brain that causes that person to not produce enough of certain chemicals, called neurotransmitters, which scientists believe are responsible for mood control. This could be compared to an illness like diabetes, where the body no longer produces enough insulin. There doesn't really have to be an outside reason. The reason is the chemical deficiency itself.

Sometimes people become depressed for what seems like a good reason—maybe they lost their job or a close friend passed away—but with clinical depression, there doesn't necessarily have to be a reason for how you feel. The chemicals in the brain which are responsible for mood control may be out of balance causing you to feel bad even though everything in your life is going well.

There Are Many Things That Can Cause Depression

The causes of depression aren't completely understood, but it is believed that the best explanation for it is that it is probably caused a combination of factors, such as an underlying genetic tendency towards the condition and certain environmental factors which can act as triggers.

Depression Is More Than Ordinary Sadness

Sadness is a part of being human, a natural reaction to painful circumstances. All of us will experience sadness at some point in our lives. Depression, however, is a physical illness with many more symptoms than an unhappy mood.

Children Are Not Immune to Depression

A myth exists that says childhood is a joyful, carefree time in our lives. While children don't experience the same problems that adults do, like work-related stress or financial pressures, this doesn't mean that they can't become depressed. Childhood brings its own unique set of stresses, such as bullying and the struggle for peer acceptance.

Depression Is a Real Illness

You are not weak or crazy. Depression is a real illness which scientists believe is caused by imbalances in certain chemicals within your brain called *neurotransmitters*. These neurotransmitters are thought to play an important role in regulating your mood as well as being involved in many other functions throughout your body.

Depression Is Treatable

You do not need to suffer if you have depression. There are several very effective treatment options available to you, including medications and psychotherapy. In addition, there are new treatments being developed all the time which are proving to be effective in cases where other treatments have failed.

Untreated Depression Is the Most Common Cause of Suicide

The proper diagnosis and treatment of depression is very important in preventing suicides. According to the Substance Abuse and Mental Health Services Association (SAMHSA), 90 percent of those who commit suicide are suffering from some sort of mental illness. And, most of these people have depression which is either undiagnosed, untreated, or undertreated.

Chapter Two

"Regular exercise such as a daily walk will reduce the likelihood of you suffering from depression"

Symptoms

What are the symptoms of depression? Depression varies from person to person, but there are some common signs and symptoms. It's important to remember that these symptoms can be part of life's normal lows. But the More symptoms you have, the stronger they are, and the longer they've lasted—the more Likely it is that you're dealing with depression.

10 common symptoms of depression:

- Feelings of helplessness and hopelessness. A bleak outlook—nothing will ever get better and there's nothing you can do to improve your situation.

- Loss of interest in daily activities. You don't care anymore about former hobbies, pastimes, social activities, or sex. You've lost your ability to feel joy and pleasure.

- Appetite or weight changes. Significant weight loss or weight gain—a change of more than 5% of body weight in a month.
- Sleep changes. Either insomnia, especially waking in the early hours of the morning, or oversleeping.

- Anger or irritability. Feeling agitated, restless, or even violent. Your tolerance level is low, your temper short, and everything and everyone gets on your nerves.

- Loss of energy. Feeling fatigued, sluggish, and physically drained. Your whole body may feel heavy, and even small tasks are exhausting or take longer to complete.

- Self-loathing. Strong feelings of worthlessness or guilt. You harshly criticize yourself for perceived faults and mistakes.

- Reckless behaviour. You engage in escapist behaviour such as substance abuse,
- compulsive gambling, reckless driving, or dangerous sports.

- Concentration problems. Trouble focusing, making decisions, or remembering
- things.

- Unexplained aches and pains. An increase in physical complaints such as
- Headaches, back pain, aching muscles, and stomach pain.

Is it depression or bipolar disorder?

Bipolar disorder, also known as manic depression, involves serious shifts in moods, energy, thinking, and behaviour. Because it looks so similar to depression when in the low phase, it is often overlooked and misdiagnosed. This can be a serious problem as taking antidepressants for bipolar depression can actually make the condition *worse*. If you've ever gone through phases where you experienced excessive feelings of euphoria, a decreased need for sleep, racing thoughts, and impulsive behaviour, consider getting evaluated for bipolar disorder.

Depression and suicide risk

Depression is a major risk factor for suicide. The deep despair and hopelessness that goes along with depression can make suicide feel like the only way to escape the pain. If you have a loved one with depression, take any suicidal talk or behaviour seriously and watch for the warning signs:

Talking about killing or harming one's self.

Expressing strong feelings of hopelessness or being trapped

An unusual preoccupation with death or dying

Acting recklessly, as if they have a death wish (e.g. speeding through red lights)

Calling or visiting people to say goodbye

Getting affairs in order (giving away prized possessions, tying up loose ends)

Saying things like "Everyone would be better off without me" or "I want out"

A sudden switch from being extremely depressed to acting calm and happy.

If you think a friend or family member is considering suicide, express your concern and seek help immediately.

If You Are Feeling Suicidal

When you're feeling depressed or suicidal, your problems don't seem temporary—they seem overwhelming and permanent. But with time, you will feel better, especially if you get help. There are many people who want to support you during this difficult time, so please reach out!

Depression causes and risk factors

While some illnesses have a specific medical cause, making treatment straight forward, depression is more complicated. Depression is not just the result of a chemical imbalance in the brain that can be simply cured with medication. It's caused by a combination of biological, sychological, and social factors. In other words, your lifestyle choices, relationships, and coping skills matter just as much—if not more so—than genetics.

Depression is a medical illness similar to diabetes or hypothyroidism, where the body does not produce enough of a needed substance to function properly. And just like these conditions, we can not simply will our bodies to make more.

It takes the correct medical intervention, such as medication, to correct the underlying chemical imbalances of depression.

Chapter Three

"Talking openly about suicidal thoughts and feelings can save a life."

What you can say

When you want to say more, but have a hard time expressing what you feel, try referencing these ten statements someone who is depressed might find helpful to hear.

"I Care"

These two simple words—"I care"—can mean so much to a person who may be feeling like the entire world is against her. A hug or a gentle touch of the hand can even get this message across. The important thing is to reach out and let the person know that she matters to you.

"I'm here for you"

Depression can feel as if no one understands what you are feeling or even cares enough to begin to understand, which can be isolating and overwhelming. When you reach out to a friend, letting them know that you are going to be there every step of the way can be very reassuring.

You may not quite know what this will look like at first, but know that just reminding your friend that you are someone he can lean on can mean the world.

"Is There Anything I Can Do to Help?"

Depression places a great weight on the person who has it, both physically and mentally, so there are probably many things you can do to ease the burden as your friend recovers.

He may be reluctant to accept your offer for fear of becoming a burden on you, so make it clear that you don't mind and want to help in the same way you know he would for you in a similar situation.

It is also possible that depression may leave your friend so tired and down that he doesn't even know what kind of help to ask for. Be prepared with a few specific suggestions, which may include:

- Could you use some help with housework or grocery shopping?
- Would you like some company for a while?

- Would you like me to drive you to your doctor appointments?

Being specific in regard to both the time and activity can be helpful. For example, instead of saying "Is there anything I can do for you?" perhaps ask, "Could I come over on Saturday morning and do some yard work for you?"

Remember, too, that the help you think your friend may need may not match with what would actually be beneficial in his eyes. Suggest—and listen.

"Have You Told Your Doctor How You Are Feeling?"

Depression treatments are a very important part of recovering from depression, but people often feel ashamed of their condition or pessimistic about whether treatment will really help.

If your friend has not yet seen a doctor, encourage him to seek help and reassure him that there is nothing wrong with asking for assistance. Depression is a real—and treatable—illness.

If he is already seeing a doctor, offer to help with picking up medications and being on time for appointments.

"Do You Need Someone to Talk With?"

Sometimes the most important thing you can do for a depressed friend is to just listen sympathetically while she talks about what is bothering her, allowing her to relieve the pressure of pent-up feelings. This can help make her mental and emotional pain more bearable as she goes through the course of treatment prescribed by her doctor and/or therapist.

Make sure to listen without interrupting. We all wish to fix things for those we care about and often offer quick fixes to cope with our own feelings of helplessness. Sometimes people who are depressed just need to talk without having the conversation taken over with well-meaning advice.

"Your Life Makes a Difference to Me"

A common feeling among those who are depressed is that their lives don't matter and no one would even care if they were gone. If you can sincerely tell your friend about all the ways that she matters to you and others, this can help her realize that she has value and worth.

"I Understand" (If You Really Do)

Before you tell someone "I understand," you should be certain that you actually do. Have you ever experienced clinical depression? If you have, it may be helpful for your friend to realize that you have experienced what he is feeling and were able to get better. Keep in mind that there are several different types of depression, and even if you did experience clinical depression, it may have been very different than what your friend is going through.

However, if what you have been through was just a mild case of the blues, your friend may feel like you are trivializing his experience by comparing it with yours. In this case, it would be best to simply admit that you don't understand exactly what he is going through, but you care about him and want to try.

Often, the best words to say are, "I don't understand, but I really want to."

"It's OK to Feel This Way"

Even though your friend's problems may seem minor to you, resist the urge to judge or come up with simple solutions. The biochemical imbalances associated with depression are what is driving how bad she feels about certain situations—not the situations themselves. Instead, let her know that you are sorry that she is feeling so badly and adopt an attitude of acceptance that this is how her depression is affecting her.

If your friend only recently started taking medications or attending counselling, it can take time for her to begin to feel better. Just as an antibiotic for a strep throat takes a while to work, antidepressants can take some time to change chemicals in the brain (sometimes upwards of eight weeks or longer). During this time, what she needs most is not references to fast, easy solutions, but an awareness that you will be by her side until her treatment works.

"You Aren't Weak or Defective"

Those who are coping with depression tend to feel weak or that there is something wrong with them. Depression may be seen as an illness to others, but those who live with it feel that it's a character flaw.

Reassure your friend that depression really is an illness caused by a biochemical imbalance in the brain, and it does not mean that he is weak. In fact, it takes a great deal of strength to fight back, so he is probably much stronger than the average person.

"There Is Hope"

While you are reassuring your friend that she has a real illness, you can also reassure her that there is hope, because, like any other medical illness, depression is treatable. Through the use of medications and therapy, she has a very good chance of returning to feeling normal again.

When Good Intentions Go Wrong

It is possible that you can say all the "right" things and your friend will still become upset with you. Each person is an individual with unique thoughts and feelings, and being angry and upset is the nature of depression. Sometimes people will lash out at those trying to help them because they are hurting and don't know where to direct those bad feelings. Whoever is nearby becomes a convenient target.

If this happens, try not to take it personally. Stay calm and continue to do what you can to love and support your friend in whatever way she will allow.

Finally, the risk of suicide is high in those suffering with depression. No matter what you say or what you do to help your friend, he may still experience suicidal thoughts and feelings. Make sure to be on the lookout for warning signs of suicide and know when to seek help.

Chapter Four

"Alternative medicine could be the way forward in treating depression"

What not to say

Knowing what to say to someone who is depressed isn't always easy. While you may feel awkward and unsure at first, know that whatever you say doesn't have to be profound or poetic. It should simply be something that comes from a place of compassion and acceptance. Try not to be dissuaded by worry over saying the "wrong" thing. Too many people with clinical depression feel alone—a state that only worsens their condition. If you don't know what to say, just say that—and tell your friend that you are there for him.

Cheer Up

In a similar vein are well-meaning exhortations to "cheer up" or "smile," as if all a depressed person needs to do to cure their depression is to decide to be happy. Just like he can't choose to "snap out it," he can't choose to "cheer up."

It Can't Be That Bad

Events that might not really bother one person may seem like insurmountable obstacles to someone with depression because they do not have the internal resources needed to cope with stressful experiences.

How bad things are in your life really has nothing to do with depression.

It's All in Your Head

Depression is caused by a deficiency in the brain of mood-regulating substances called neurotransmitters.

While technically the deficiency of mood-regulating substances is occurring "in your head," depression is a very real illness.

Who Cares?

Depression can make a person feel as if they have no worth as a human being.

The worst thing you can do is to confirm these feelings for him by saying that nobody cares.

Stop Feeling Sorry for Yourself

A person with depression is not choosing to feel sorry for himself. It is the result of a chemical imbalance in the brain.

How he feels is not a choice at all; it is a chemical imbalance he has no control over.

It's Your Own Fault

While we do not entirely understand the causes of depression, we do know for certain that no one chooses to have this painful condition. Instead, it is believed by scientists to be at least in part an inherited condition passed along to us by our ancestors.

In addition to being hereditary, certain environmental factors may also play a role, perhaps by triggering any underlying inherited vulnerability to depression.

You Understand (When You Really Don't)

It's very easy to say that you understand what another person is going through, but if you've never truly experienced clinical depression, then it may feel to him like you are minimizing what he is experiencing. There is simply no comparison between a mild case of the blues and clinical depression. While your mild depression quickly passed, he sees no end in sight for his suffering.

Rather than saying that you understand, it would better to say that you don't understand, but you care about him and would like to try.

It Could Be Worse

It may well be true that a person's life could be worse, but depression isn't about how bad things are; it's about how bad they feel for the person at that moment.

You Never Think of Anybody but Yourself

While it may seem like a depressed person is very wrapped up in his own life, it doesn't mean he is selfish or unconcerned about others.

When a person feels the intense pain and sadness associated with depression, it becomes very difficult to focus on anything but that pain.

But You Don't Look Depressed

People with depression can become very good at putting on a fake smile and going through the motions of everyday life. This does not mean, however, that they are not falling apart inside.

You Just Need to Try Harder

Because depression is an invisible illness, it doesn't always show just hard a person is already trying. Hearing someone tell you that you just need to try harder when you are already giving it your best effort can be both frustrating and insulting.

You Should Get Out More

Unfortunately, the symptoms of depression, such as fatigue and lack of motivation, are probably what are causing him to stay home in the first place.

If he felt well enough to go out, then he wouldn't be depressed.

You think you've Got It Bad

Avoid turning it into a competition for who is feeling worse. This makes the other person feel like you are minimizing their pain and not really listening to what they have to say.

This too shall pass

While this may be true, it is not helpful to a depressed person to hear this. It's just too vague a statement to offer any real hope. When will his depression pass? Will it be days? Weeks? Months? Years?

This statement simply provides no comfort to a person who is suffering and has no idea when they will begin to feel better, if ever.

Chapter Five

"Your life is precious and does matter"

Treatment

The good news is that because it is a biologically-based illness, it is also very treatable.

The most commonly-used treatments for depression are antidepressant. Combined therapy is considered to be the most effective. For most people, these treatments will be enough to achieve relief from their depression symptoms. In some cases, however, medication and psychotherapy are not effective.

Medication

Antidepressants work to normalize naturally occurring brain chemicals called neurotransmitters, notably serotonin and norepinephrine. Other antidepressants work on the neurotransmitter Dopamine.

Scientists studying depression have found that particular chemicals are involved in regulating mood, but they are unsure of the exact ways in which they work. Medication should be stopped only under a doctor's supervision. Some medications need to be gradually stopped to give the body time to adjust. Although antidepressants are not habit-forming or addictive, abruptly ending an antidepressant can cause withdrawal symptoms or lead to a relapse. Some individuals, such as those with chronic or recurrent depression, may need to stay on the Medication indefinitely.

In addition, if one medication does not work, patients should be open to trying another. Patients who did not get well after taking a first medication Increased their chances of becoming symptom-free after they switched to a different medication or added another medication to their existing one. Sometimes stimulants, anti-anxiety medications, or other medications are used in conjunction with an antidepressant, especially if the patient has a co-existing mental or physical

disorder. However, neither anti-anxiety edications nor stimulants
Are effective against depression when taken alone, and both should be taken only under a doctor's close supervision.

What are the side effects of antidepressants?

Antidepressants may cause mild and often temporary side effects in some people, but they are usually not long-term.

However, any unusual reactions or side effects that interfere with normal functioning should be reported to a doctor immediately.

Alternative Medicine

Many of the products such as oils and teas that are formulated from natural products have diverse and multi - purpose roles especially in the treatment of depression.

Countries such as Canada and some states in the USA are starting to legalise and recognize these natural products for medicinal use. Cannabis has become a multi- billion dollar industry. The following plants have healing qualities and I recommend researching or consulting with your doctor them before using them.

Cannabis

Moringa

Maroela

Complementary Therapies

Reflexology

Body stress relieve

Therapeutic massage

Aroma Therapy

Yoga

Meditation

Chapter Six

"There are three deaths. The first is when the body ceases to function. The second is when the body is consigned to the grave. The third is that moment, sometime in the future, when your name is spoken for the last time."

Three Deaths

I was having an intellectual conversation with a likeminded friend around the kitchen table. Gerhardt is a lot younger than me but is filled with the wisdom of an ancient person. We were discussing depression and trying to understand it better. The conversation was incredibly interesting because we could not believe how likeminded we were and have the same values and thoughts on humanity. People are often afraid to openly say what they are thinking in fear of the implications and ramifications of doing just that.

Realizing we were comfortable of discussing our thoughts we found that we had a lot of common theories.

The conversation had lead us to legacies that we leave behind.

He mentioned that there is a belief somewhere in Mexico that we all die three deaths, a statement that was so profound that I felt I had to write about it. The first time we die is the day when we realize that we can get physically hurt as a child and death can become a reality so we become more careful and aware of our physical abilities. This normally happens in early childhood where we did not know that it was possible to die. It could also be when we have a direct association with death when someone dies that is close to you, e.g. a grandparent or family member. Naturally in today's times we are exposed to death all the time by different mediums such as the movies and news documentaries. This first statement did not rattle me but I continued to listen to what is being said.

The second death is the day we actually die. Which is common sense but it was the last death that had me thinking.

The third death we experience is the day when your name is mentioned for the last time by anyone on this earth…………what a profound statement!

It leads me to conclude that your life is precious and does matter. You do make a difference.

Epilogue

If this handbook helps just one person or saves one life then the purpose of the book has served its purpose. Many people don't even know they are depressed. I know what it is to be depressed which has led me to formulate a few theories which I hope to substantiate through research one day.

Intelligent people commit suicide from over contemplating on an universal or global level. Depression causes unexplained physical pain.

A healthy life style with a regular exercise such as walking is more than likely going you to enjoy a healthier mind.

Contribution and thanks

I would like to thank the following people that helped me develop this handbook on depression.

Gerhard Nieuwoudt – Life coach

Renata Roos – Therapeutic Reflexologist

Bryan C. Price – Author

www.ingramcontent.com/pod-product-compliance
Lightning Source LLC
Chambersburg PA
CBHW080845170526
45158CB00009B/2642